Wheat Belly Box Set

Wheat Belly Recipes & Gluten Free Slow Cooker Recipes

Table of Contents

Introduction

This book contains more than 30 delicious wheat-free recipes that adhere to the principles of the Wheat Belly Diet program, which the respected American cardiologist and New York Times best-selling author Dr. William Davis introduced in 2011. It is a system of eating that encourages the use of organic, wheat-free foods to help achieve an ideal weight and heal the body from illness.

All of the recipes in this book use ingredients that are gluten-free, low in sodium and contain zero traces of refined sugar. This means that you can now enjoy scrumptious breakfasts, soups, salads, main dishes and desserts without adding inches to your waistline.

Apart from the nutrient-dense Wheat Belly recipes, you will find in this book essential information about Dr. Davis' Wheat Belly Diet program, including its principles, food list, benefits and coping mechanisms that will keep you focused on your journey towards self-improvement and complete wellness.

Moreover, this book will effectively guide you towards healthier cooking by showing you wheat-free substitutes to common ingredients. Becoming aware of healthier options that are available in the market increases your chance of using them in the kitchen and obtaining a grain-free lifestyle.

In addition second book contains 40 mouth-watering, gluten free dishes that are simple and easy to prepare, thanks to the wonderful features of a slow cooker.

Gluten free eating has become a priority among today's health-conscious members of society. With the current rise in the number of people acquiring celiac disease, cancer, irritable bowel syndrome, food allergies and other health problems, medical research has determined that wheat products play a major part in this unhealthy cycle of illness. This discovery has led doctors and nutrition experts to encourage people to adopt a gluten free lifestyle wherein healthier, organic meals without wheat products should be consumed to achieve balance within the mind, body and spirit.

To help us achieve more balance in our health, this book provides gluten free recipes that we can incorporate in our daily meal preparation. The ingredients used in each dish are 100% gluten free and is cooked to perfection with the use of a slow cooker. We will also see how interesting gluten free cooking can be with the colorful mix of fruits, vegetables, dairy and meats found in each slow cooker meal. The dishes are easy to make and tasty that you might just get hooked on using the slow cooker every day.

Let's begin the journey.

Wheat Belly Recipes – Simple And Delicious Wheat Belly Recipes To Lose Weight For Beginners

Chapter 1: Wheat Belly Diet: Lose the Grains to Lose the Gut

"Wheat is a silent killer and a silent disrupter of health, in addition to causing myriad overt symptoms of health disruption."

Dr. William Davis, M.D.
Cardiologist and N.Y. Times best-selling author

The Wheat Belly Diet, a groundbreaking health program developed by American cardiologist and author Dr. William Davis, promotes a grain-free way of eating that will help lose unwanted pounds and shed unhealthy visceral fat. Based on actual testimonials found in Dr. Davis' website, people who have undergone this diet program have lost more than 10 pounds in 7 days and are gradually winning their lifelong battle with the bulge.

However, more than being an effective weight loss tool, the Wheat Belly program aims at helping reverse the symptoms of serious medical conditions such as obesity, diabetes, autoimmune disease, celiac disease and mental disorders. It is a complete wellness venture that will rid the body of the effects of modern grains, sugars and processed foods, leaving a healthier and lighter physique.

Here is an overview of this life-changing diet program:

The Dangers of Modern Wheat and Gluten

The Wheat Belly concept was introduced by Dr. Davis in his 2011 New York Times best-selling book *Wheat Belly*. The book reveals that food products made from modern wheat, also referred to as *Frankenwheat*, are not only toxic, but also trigger hormones within the body that increase addictive behavior. For this reason, people have become fond of eating wheat-based foods such as breads, pasta, pastries and grains without being mindful of portion control.

Gluten, the main component of genetically-modified wheat, is a protein that elicits wheat addiction and other health problems upon its entry into the stomach. Once a person ingests gluten-rich foods, the immune system attacks the protein and damages the intestinal walls in the process. Cell damage creates entry points for bacteria and other foreign entities into the bloodstream; hence, causing disease and hormonal imbalance.

Note also that apart from causing disease, gluten can also trigger weight gain. Processed and genetically-modified foods that contain wheat are typically high in calories and contain loads of sugar, sodium and bad carbohydrates. For this reason, regular wheat product consumption results to a high and unhealthy Body Mass Index (BMI) and unsightly excess fat in the mid-section.

Moreover, people with high BMIs increase their chances of acquiring lifestyle diseases such as obesity, type 2 Diabetes and heart disease.

The dangerous effects of gluten have triggered the public's interest to develop gluten-free diet programs that will address the needs of people who have become overweight and sick. A great development in modern nutrition is the Wheat Belly Diet, which promotes healthy, organic eating amidst the rise of junk food and instant meals within the food industry.

Wheat Belly vs. Gluten Free

The Wheat Belly program is a plant and animal-based diet inspired by the combined principles of Paleo and gluten-free diets. The main purpose of this diet program is to encourage people to eat and drink organic while avoiding all wheat products, sugars and processed foods. This very restrictive diet requires discipline and meal preparation in order to reap its long-term health benefits.

Food and beverage that are allowed on the Wheat Belly diet include vegetables, fruits, eggs, poultry, meat, seafood, herbs, spices, healthy oils, water, herbal teas, and black coffee. You can eat dairy products, seeds and soy products, but in limited portions. On the other hand, it is necessary to avoid grains, processed food, junk food, sugars and artificial drinks at all cost. However, most importantly, you need to avoid products marketed as gluten-free versions of pastas, sauces and baking products.

Although the Wheat Belly Diet promotes gluten-free eating, it strongly discourages people to buy foods such as gluten-free pasta or gluten-free flours. According to Dr. Davis, pre-packaged gluten-free products are made of ingredients loaded with bad carbohydrates such as potatoes, rice and corn. This is why people who eat gluten-free versions of grains and processed snacks tend to gain more weight and experience surges in their blood-sugar levels.

The key to a successful Wheat Belly Diet is to eat natural foods filled with vitamins, minerals, fiber, protein and good carbohydrates. There are no shortcuts to achieving your ideal weight, so choose to eat organic and wheat-free and be disciplined enough to maintain this lifestyle.

Luckily, this book contains 32 easy Wheat Belly recipes that you can whip up in your own kitchen. These dishes are high in nutrients, low in calories and contain zero traces of wheat, which will guarantee you a healthy weight loss of 3-5 pounds per week. This program will make you lighter, more energetic and less susceptible to disease. As a matter of fact, it may be the diet that will help eliminate your weight and health problems forever.

The succeeding chapters will answer your Wheat Belly questions in a more in-depth manner and show you how simple it is to create flavorful and nutritious meals that adhere to the Wheat Belly diet principles.

Enjoy cooking wheat-free dishes and embrace a lighter and healthier you!

Chapter 2: Top 10 Frequently Asked Questions

"The easiest diet is, you know, eat vegetables, eat fresh food. Just a really sensible diet like you read about all the time."

Drew Carey

The Wheat Belly Diet is an effective program that will help you reach your goal weight, lose belly fat and achieve optimum health. Here are answers to Wheat Belly's burning questions that will reveal essential information about the program:

1. What is the main principle of the Wheat Belly Diet?

   The Wheat Belly Diet is based on the principle that wheat and wheat-based products such as processed foods, junk carbohydrates and refined sugars are toxic for the body. These types of foods are the culprits of visceral fat, which ultimately leads to obesity and disease. Thus, Wheat Belly advocates to follow a plant and animal-based diet wherein the foods are healthier and closest to their natural state.

2. Is the Wheat Belly Diet a weight-loss program?

   This grain-free diet is useful in losing weight. As a matter of fact, eliminating wheat from regular meals will slash more than 300 calories from your daily caloric intake. Lesser calories will later result to weight loss and a slimmer body.

   However, Wheat Belly is more than just the typical weight-loss program: it is a positive lifestyle change that benefits the stomach, immune system and hormones by supplying them with amino acids that keep them healthy and fully functioning. In the end, our bodies become lighter, slimmer and more importantly, disease-free.

3. How is wheat harmful to the body?

Wheat-based foods contain gluten, a protein that is useful in making bread soft and chewy. Once gluten enters the stomach, its sub-protein gliadin triggers abnormal immune response and allows healthy cells in the intestines to be attacked by antibodies. The damage in the intestinal wall leads to inflammation and disease.

Another harmful effect of processed wheat products is weight gain. Pasta, rice, breads and pastries contain lots of calories from empty carbohydrates, sugar, sodium and unhealthy fat. Eating wheat products regularly can cause inflammation or bloating in the stomach, higher blood sugar levels and inability to lose weight.

4. What foods can I eat on the Wheat Belly Diet?

- Vegetables – Sweet potatoes, zucchini, whole corn, avocadoes, jicama, artichokes, bell peppers, carrots, squash, cauliflower, garlic, peas, onions, shallots, lettuce, spinach, leeks, tomatoes, broccoli, turnip, eggplant, kale, cucumber, mushrooms, chili peppers, scallions, cabbage, spinach, green beans, asparagus

- Fruits (in moderation) – Lemons, cranberries, blueberries, strawberries, cherries, raspberries, limes, blackberries, apple, orange, pear, apricot, grapes, pineapple, mango, banana

- Dairy – Egg, cream, cheeses such as cheddar, Monterey Jack, Parmesan, ricotta, Swiss, Gruyere, Romano, mozzarella, cottage and cream, Greek yoghurt, sour cream, organic butter, buttermilk, half and half

- Organic meat and poultry – Pork, beef, lamb, chicken, buffalo, duck, veal, turkey, quail, bacon, Italian sausage

- Seafood – Shrimp, crab, lobster, oyster, tuna, salmon, cod, squid, halibut, tilapia, clams, mahi mahi, swordfish, mussels, snapper

- Legumes (in moderation) – Kidney beans, lima beans, pinto beans, black beans, chickpeas, black-eyed peas, lentils

- Herbs and spices – Basil, tarragon, sage, thyme, rosemary, dill, mint, parsley, cilantro, bay leaf, oregano, chili powder, ginger, turmeric, paprika, onion powder, mustard, cumin, star anise, cinnamon, nutmeg, allspice, ground pepper, whole peppercorns, salt, wasabi

- Condiments – Coconut aminos, fish sauce, hot sauce, mirin, vinegars, horseradish, tapenades, mustards

- Baking products – Nut butters, semi-sweet chocolate chips, almond flour, chickpea flour, ground flaxseed, walnut meal, coconut flour, hazelnut meal, stevia, vanilla extract, baking soda, cream of tartar, baking powder, cocoa powder, xantham gum, active dry yeast

- Nuts and seeds – Walnuts, cashews, almonds, hazelnuts, pecans, sesame seeds, pumpkin seeds, flaxseeds, sunflower seeds

- Fats – Coconut oil, olive oil, avocado oil, walnut oil, flaxseed oil

- Cooking products – Green curry paste, tomato juice, tomato paste, homemade broth, coconut milk, fermented and pickled vegetables, shredded coconut, coconut flakes

- Drinks – Water, black coffee, almond milk, herbal tea, fruit-infused water, freshly-squeezed or blended fruit juice (preferably fruits with low sugar and high water content), natural smoothies, coconut water, red wine

5. What foods are prohibited?

- Gluten grains – Wheat, rye, faro, spelt, kamut, durum, barley, triticale

- Baking flours - Whole wheat, all purpose, rice, potato, tapioca, quinoa, teff, amaranth, millet, tapioca

- Processed meats - Ham, sausages, pepperoni, salami

- Cheeses - Gorgonzola, Roquefort and blue cheese

- Wheat products - Breakfast cereals, crepes, noodles, pasta, breads, pies, cookies, waffles, beignets, pita bread, wraps, pancakes, burrito, cupcakes, baguette

- Unhealthy oils – Margarine, sunflower oil, grapeseed oil, soybean oil, canola oil, corn oil

- Cooking products - Breadcrumbs, bacon bits, croutons, ramen, gnocchi, cornstarch, matzo, roux, tabbouleh, gravy, hydrolyzed vegetable protein, orzo, curry powder, seasoning mixes, soup and stock base, soy meat

- Beverages – Beer, flavored coffee, vodka, wine coolers, milk teas, soda, artificial fruit juices, milkshakes

- Sweets and snacks – Energy bars, chewing gum, jelly beans, chocolate bars, dried fruit, ice cream, potato chips, roasted peanuts, jams, trail mixes, jellies, puddings, frosting, fast food burgers, hotdogs, fries, pies

- Sweeteners – Honey, sugar, agave nectar, corn syrup, maple syrup, sucrose

- Condiments – Ketchup, soy sauce, salad dressings, miso, teriyaki sauce

6. What are the benefits of undergoing the Wheat Belly program?

The Wheat Belly Diet is a program that does not include confusing stages, calorie counting or special food items that are hard to find. Once you see the Wheat Belly recipes found in this book, you will realize how easy it is to create delicious meals while in the process of losing pounds.

Apart from weight loss, the organic ingredients in a Wheat Belly diet such as vegetables, fruits and protein help lower blood sugar, cholesterol and blood pressure, as well as prevent the onset of medical conditions such as heart ailments, cataracts, allergies, celiac disease, arthritis and cancer, among others.

7. What are the disadvantages of the Wheat Belly program?

Losing 30 pounds in 12 weeks is achievable with the Wheat Belly lifestyle. However, this program takes a lot of discipline and willpower given the presence of wheat products all around us. It also doesn't help that food labels contain very fine print about the gluten content of foods, so we need to read food labels carefully.

In addition, beginners may experience wheat withdrawals within a few days of giving up grains. Unpleasant symptoms may include nausea, constipation, intense cravings and emotional imbalance. Taking iron and magnesium supplements may do the trick, or relaxation techniques such as meditation or self-affirmation exercises may help calm down your anxiety.

8. Will going on the Wheat Belly make me hungry?

Grains and processed foods may seem heavy on the stomach, but these are all empty calories. On the other hand, the Wheat Belly food list contains nutritious ingredients that are high in vitamins, protein, fiber and good carbohydrates. This implies that organic foods such as steamed vegetables or roasted chicken can fill up the stomach and prevent unnecessary cravings.

9. Why am I not losing weight in the Wheat Belly program?

A major cause of weight gain while undergoing a gluten-free diet such as the Wheat Belly program is consuming wheat products labeled as "gluten-free." These so-called gluten free pastas and pastries may contain more sugar and carbohydrates than their whole grain counterparts, which makes them more harmful for human consumption.

It is also advisable to combine exercise with the Wheat Belly diet. This will help speed up metabolism and burn more calories.

10 Where can I find Wheat Belly recipes?

The following chapters include mouth-watering yet healthy recipes that follow the principles of the Wheat Belly lifestyle. You will realize how easy it is to forego wheat by creating delectable dishes using fresh, wheat-free ingredients.

Start your disease-free, grain-free lifestyle by trying out the recipes in this book. These Wheat Belly dishes will not only help you lose inches, but it will also provide you with a pain-free and worry-free existence that only organic produce can give.

Chapter 3: Wheat Belly Breakfast and Brunch Recipes

Pink Sunrise Smoothie

Begin the day with a fruity breakfast smoothie that will give your body the vitamins and fiber that it needs.

Serves: 2

Ready in: 10 minutes

Ingredients:

- 3 tablespoons Greek yoghurt

- 2 peaches, pitted and diced

- 1 cup natural pomegranate juice

- 1 ½ teaspoons liquid stevia

- 2 tablespoons flaxseed oil

- 6 ice cubes

Procedure:

1. Place yoghurt, peaches, pomegranate juice, stevia, flaxseed oil and ice cubes in a blender and process for 2 minutes. Pour the smoothie into glasses and serve immediately.

Hi-Fiber Hash Browns

Apples, sweet potatoes and almond meal make up this fiber-enriched dish that is best served with a sunny side up egg.

Serves: 4

Ready in: 1 hour

Ingredients:

- Pinch of salt and pepper

- 2 apples, peeled, cored and shredded

- 2 sweet potatoes, peeled and grated

- ½ cup almond meal

- 1 teaspoon garlic powder

- 1¼ cup olive oil

Procedure:

1. Place shredded apples and sweet potatoes in a bowl and fill it up with water. Soak them for 30 minutes then squeeze the pulp to drain out the moisture.

2. Transfer the drained fruit into another bowl and add in the almond meal, ¼ cup olive oil, salt, pepper and garlic powder. Mix well then form 8 thin hash browns from the mixture.

3. Heat the remaining olive oil in a pan over medium-high flame. Place the hash browns on the pan and cook each side for 3 minutes. Place the cooked hash browns in a plate and serve hot.

Chicken and Greens Frittata

A serving of this delicious, vegetable-filled frittata will help boost your energy and metabolism throughout the day.

Serves: 4

Ready in: 30 minutes

Ingredients:

- 6 whole eggs
- ½ cup grated Parmesan cheese
- ½ cup shredded leftover chicken meat
- 1 teaspoon dried dill
- ½ cup frozen spinach, chopped
- 4 green onions, chopped
- Pinch of sea salt and ground black pepper
- 2 tablespoons olive oil

Procedure:

1. Preheat the oven to 425°F.

2. Whisk together eggs, salt, pepper and dill. Set this aside.

3. Heat the olive oil in a skillet over medium-high flame. Add in the green onions, spinach and chicken then cook for 3 minutes. Pour the egg mixture in and leave it to set for 3-4 minutes.

4. Once the eggs are set, sprinkle cheese on top of the dish then transfer the pan into the oven. Let the frittata cook for 7 minutes. Once the frittata is ready, let it cool at room temperature before placing on a serving plate. Serve warm.

Breakfast Cabbage Bowl with Carrots and Peppers

Cook some shredded cabbage in olive oil then season it with salt and spices: this is a low-calorie and wheat-free substitute to unhealthy fried rice.

Serves: 2

Ready in: 20 minutes

Ingredients:

- 4 cups finely shredded cabbage

- 1 tablespoon organic butter

- 1 red onion, minced

- 2 garlic cloves, crushed

- 1 cup shredded carrot

- 1 red bell pepper, deseeded and cut into thin strips

- ½ teaspoon ginger powder

- Pinch of sea salt

Procedure:

1. Heat the butter in a pan over medium-high flame. Toss in the garlic and onion, cover the pan and cook the ingredients for 3

minutes. Add the cabbage and stir. Cover the pan and let the cabbage simmer for 3 minutes.

2. Remove the cover then sprinkle sea salt and ginger powder on the cabbage. Adjust the heat of the stovetop to high then continue cooking for 3 minutes or until the cabbage has dried up. Finally, add in the bell pepper and carrots and let the dish cook for 2 more minutes.

3. Transfer the dish into individual bowls and serve while hot.

Grain-Free Breakfast Loaf

This recipe uses a mixture of almond and coconut flours for a low-sugar, gluten free loaf that won't harm the gut.

Serves: 6

Ready in: 50 minutes

Ingredients:

- 2 ripe bananas, mashed
- 1 cup almond flour
- 3 eggs
- ¼ cup coconut flour
- ½ teaspoon salt
- 1 teaspoon baking soda
- 1 teaspoon liquid stevia
- 2 teaspoons vanilla
- 1 teaspoon cinnamon
- 2 tablespoons coconut oil
- ¼ cup dark chocolate chips

- ½ teaspoon nutmeg

Procedure:

1. Preheat the oven to 350°F and line a loaf pan with parchment paper.

2. In a small bowl, whisk together the eggs, coconut oil, vanilla, stevia and bananas. Set this aside.

3. In another bowl, blend together the almond flour, coconut flour, baking soda, nutmeg, salt and cinnamon. Slowly fold in the banana mixture into the dry ingredients and mix well. Finally, blend in the chocolate chips.

4. Pour the batter into the lined loaf pan and place it in the oven. Bake the loaf for 40 minutes. Let it cool at room temperature before serving.

Grain-Free Breakfast Cake

This recipe will show you how easy it is to cook a healthy breakfast: just whisk the ingredients in a bowl and cook it in a microwave.

Servings: 1

Ready in: 5 minutes

Ingredients:

- 1 banana, peeled and chopped
- 1 whole egg
- 1 drop vanilla extract
- 1 tablespoon melted organic butter
- 2 tablespoons almond flour
- ¼ teaspoon baking soda
- ¼ teaspoon cinnamon powder
- 1 tablespoon water
- 2 tablespoons light coconut milk
- 1 drop liquid stevia
- Banana slices for garnish

Procedure:

1. In a microwaveable bowl, whisk together the almond flour, water, butter, egg, baking soda, vanilla, coconut milk, stevia and cinnamon powder. Mix the ingredients well.

2. Place the bowl in a microwave. Set the temperature to high then microwave the dish for 2 minutes. If the mixture still seems raw, add another 30 seconds of cooking time. Take out the bowl and let the pancake cool at room temperature for 5 minutes. Top the dish with a few banana slices.

Chapter 4: Wheat Belly Soup Recipes

Spicy Carrot Soup

Carrots contain a high level of Vitamin A, which promotes cell formation, healthy eyesight and normal immune system activities.

Serves: 4

Ready in: 30 minutes

Ingredients:

- 6 cups chopped carrots
- 2 teaspoons chopped parsley
- ½ cup water
- 3 cups homemade vegetable broth
- 1 small onion, minced
- 2 teaspoons cayenne pepper
- 1 teaspoon olive oil

Procedure:

1. Heat the oil in a soup pot over medium-high flame. Add the onions and cook until it becomes translucent. Next, add the cayenne pepper, carrots then stir. Pour the broth into the pot, cover it then allow the mixture to simmer for 15 minutes.

2. After 15 minutes, pour the hot soup in a blender then add the parsley. Slightly cover the blender then process it for 1 minute or until the soup becomes smooth. Place the soup back into the pot then add water. Mix it well before serving.

Homemade Cream of Asparagus

A hearty bowl of this light yet flavorful asparagus soup contains blood sugar-friendly vitamins such as iron, chromium, magnesium and folate.

Serves: 4

Ready in: 40 minutes

Ingredients:

- 450 grams fresh asparagus, trimmed and chopped
- 1 white onion, minced
- 1 ½ cup homemade chicken broth
- ½ cup coconut milk
- 2 tablespoons organic butter
- Pinch of garlic powder
- Pinch of salt

Procedure:

1. Place the butter and onions in a saucepan over medium-high flame and cook for 5 minutes while stirring. Once the onions are translucent, add in the asparagus, garlic powder, salt,

chicken broth and coconut milk. Lower the heat to medium and bring the soup to a simmer. Cook for 10 minutes.

2. After 10 minutes, turn off the heat then pour the soup into a blender. Pulse the mixture 2 to 3 times until a creamy texture is produced. Serve immediately.

Smoked Vegetables Soup

The oven-roasted tomatoes, peppers and zucchinis provide a smoky flavor that makes this soup uniquely flavorful.

Serves: 5

Ready in: 1 hour

Ingredients:

- ½ cup cherry tomatoes
- 1 red bell pepper, trimmed, deseeded and chopped
- 1 green bell pepper, trimmed, deseeded and chopped
- 1 small red onion, quartered
- 1 zucchini, sliced
- ½ cup chopped cabbage
- 4 cups homemade chicken broth
- 1 teaspoon chopped basil
- ¼ cup olive oil
- Pinch of sea salt and pepper

Procedure:

1. Preheat the oven to 400°F and prepare a baking pan.

2. Mix the tomatoes, peppers, onions and zucchini in the baking pan and season with salt and pepper. Drizzle olive oil over the vegetables and toss. Place the vegetables in the oven and roast them for 20 minutes.

3. Place the roasted vegetables in a medium saucepan and add in the cabbage, basil and chicken broth. Cover it then let the soup simmer over medium flame for 20 minutes. Pour the mixture into a blender then process for 1 minute. Serve immediately or let it cool before placing in the freezer.

Dairy-Free Cream of Mushroom

If you love canned cream of mushroom, then you will appreciate this healthier version that uses shiitake mushrooms cooked in spices and white wine.

Serves: 3

Ready in: 30 minutes

Ingredients:

- 1 cup sliced shiitake mushrooms
- 3 cups water
- ¼ cup white wine
- ½ white onion, minced
- 2 tablespoons olive oil
- 2 teaspoons grass-fed butter
- 2 thyme sprigs
- 2 garlic cloves, crushed
- Pinch of sea salt and ground black pepper

Procedure:

1. Heat the oil in a soup pot over medium-high heat. Add in the mushrooms and cook for 3 minutes. Remove the mushrooms and set this aside.

2. In the same pot, add in the garlic and onions and cook for 8 minutes. Once the onions are translucent, add in the thyme and white wine. Scrape the mushroom drippings inside the pot while simmering the mixture.

3. Pour in the water and cover the pot. Simmer the soup for 15 minutes.

4. Place the cooked mushrooms and soup in the blender and process for 1 minute. For a chunkier soup, pulse the mixture once or twice then serve immediately.

Parmesan Cauliflower Soup

Store this anti-inflammatory vegetable soup inside the freezer for weeks and have a ready-to-eat meal that's light and cheesy.

Serves: 4

Ready in: 1 hour 15 minutes

Ingredients:

- 1 cauliflower head, cut into florets
- ½ cup water
- 2 tablespoons grass-fed butter
- 2 tablespoons olive oil
- 4 cups homemade chicken stock
- 1 onion, chopped
- 1 teaspoon sea salt
- ½ teaspoon white pepper

Procedure:

1. Preheat the oven to 375°F and prepare a small baking dish.

2. Rub the olive oil on the cauliflower florets and place them in the baking dish. Pour water into the dish and season the vegetables with salt. Place the cauliflower in the oven and bake for 45 minutes or until the vegetable is tender when poked with a knife.

3. Once the cauliflower is tender, remove it from the oven and let it cool for 5 minutes. Chop the vegetables and set aside.

4. Heat the butter in a soup pot placed over medium-high flame. Add in onions and cook for 5 minutes. Blend in the chopped cauliflower and pour the stock into the pot. Season the mixture with pepper then cover it. Simmer the soup for 10 minutes.

5. Pour the boiling mixture into a blender and process until smooth. Place the soup back into the pot and simmer before serving.

Chapter 5: Wheat Belly Salad Recipes

Tangy Grilled Apple and Watercress Salad

This vitamin-packed plate of healthy fruit and vegetables will help fill the stomach with the right amount of carbohydrates and fiber.

Serves: 2

Ready in: 30 minutes

Ingredients:

- 2 green apples, cored and sliced into wedges

- 3 cups watercress leaves

- 2 tablespoons fresh orange juice

- 1 drop liquid stevia

- ½ cup toasted almonds, chopped

- 1 tablespoon apple cider vinegar

- 1 teaspoon ground mustard

- 1 teaspoon olive oil

- 2 tablespoons grated Cheddar cheese

- Pinch of salt

Procedure:

1. In a small bowl, whisk together the orange juice, stevia, vinegar, salt, mustard and olive oil until a smooth vinaigrette is formed. Set this aside.

2. Place the apple wedges on a grill pan over medium-low heat and grill each side of the fruit for 3 minutes.

3. Assemble your salad by placing the watercress leaves and vinaigrette in a salad bowl and tossing them together. Arrange the grilled apples on top of the salad. Serve the dish with a sprinkle of almonds and cheese.

Grapefruit Avocado Salad

This refreshing and juicy salad contains high doses of Vitamin C, potassium, carbohydrates and healthy fats that help strengthen the immune system.

Serves: 3

Ready in: 20 minutes

Ingredients:

- 3 cups red grapefruit sections
- 1 avocado, peeled, pitted and chopped
- 2 tablespoons lime juice
- ½ red onion, sliced
- 1 tablespoon olive oil
- 2 tablespoons fresh mint
- 1 tablespoon freshly-chopped parsley
- Pinch of sea salt and ground black pepper

Procedure:

1. In a small bowl, whisk together oil, lime juice, salt and pepper. Set this aside.

2. Toss together the grapefruit, avocado, mint, onion and parsley in a salad bowl. Drizzle the lime vinaigrette on the salad and mix well. Place the salad in the fridge for 10 minutes. Serve cold.

Creamy Romaine Salad with Berries

Dressing is not necessary when eating this refreshing salad: the creamy avocado meat gives flavor and texture to the fruits and greens.

Serves: 2

Ready in: 20 minutes

Ingredients:

- 1 avocado, peeled, pitted and mashed

- 6 strawberries, trimmed and halved

- ½ cup blueberries

- 1 tablespoon extra-virgin olive oil

- 1 teaspoon salt

- 1 teaspoon ground black pepper

- 1 teaspoon toasted sesame seeds

- 1 tablespoon chopped almonds

- Half a head of romaine lettuce, roughly torn

Procedure:

1. Place the mashed avocado, salt, pepper and olive in a salad bowl and whisk them together.

2. Add in the lettuce, strawberries and blueberries. Toss the ingredients together. Sprinkle the sesame seeds and almonds on top of the salad. Place the dish in the fridge for at least 10 minutes before serving.

Baked Zucchini and Sweet Potato Salad

Zucchini and sweet potatoes contain gut-friendly minerals and good carbohydrates that will keep you satiated and free from cravings.

Serves: 3

Ready in: 20 minutes

Ingredients:

- 1 zucchini, sliced thinly

- 1 small sweet potato, sliced thinly

- 1 tablespoon olive oil

- 3 garlic cloves, minced

- ¼ teaspoon sea salt

- 1 teaspoon lime juice

- Pinch of ground black pepper

Procedure:

1. Preheat the oven to 375°F and line a baking sheet with parchment paper. Arrange the sliced potatoes and zucchini on

the baking sheet and place it in the oven. Bake the vegetables for 10-12 minutes. Set this aside.

2. While the vegetables are baking, heat half of the olive oil in a pan over medium flame. Add in the garlic and cook until golden brown. Let the garlic cool and set it aside.

3. In a small bowl, whisk together the remaining olive oil, salt, black pepper and lime juice and set aside.

4. Take out the vegetables from the oven and arrange them on a serving plate. Sprinkle the toasted garlic on top of the vegetables then drizzle the lime dressing on top of it. Serve immediately.

Spicy Asparagus Salad

Liven up your weight loss routine by having a serving of this spicy and sweet salad made of raw asparagus, lettuce and onions.

Serves: 4

Ready in: 20 minutes

Ingredients:

- 1 bunch raw asparagus, trimmed and shredded into thin ribbons
- 1 small red onion, sliced thinly
- 3 scallions, chopped
- 2 cups shredded lettuce
- 1 garlic clove, crushed
- 2 mint leaves, chopped
- 1/3 cup chopped hazelnuts
- 2 tablespoons olive oil
- 1 teaspoon sesame oil
- 1 tablespoon apple cider vinegar
- 1 tablespoon lime juice

- 2 teaspoons chili powder

- ½ teaspoon powdered ginger

- 1 drop of liquid stevia

- Pinch of sea salt and pepper

Procedure:

1. To make the dressing, whisk together the oils, vinegar, lime juice, chili powder, ginger, stevia, garlic, salt and pepper until smooth.

2. Mix together the asparagus, onions, scallions, mint leaves and lettuce leaves in a salad bowl. Pour in the dressing and toss them altogether. Sprinkle the hazelnuts on top before serving.

Chapter 6: Wheat Belly Meat Recipes

Wheat Belly Pepper Steak

Have a hearty and highly-nutritious meal with this grilled steak entrée served with a pepper and onion gravy.

Serves: 4

Ready in: 30 minutes

Ingredients:

- 500 grams flank steak, halved

- 1 tablespoon olive oil

- ¾ cup tomato puree

- ½ teaspoon liquid stevia

- ½ teaspoon chili powder

- 1 tablespoon paprika

- 1 teaspoon ground black pepper

- ½ teaspoon oregano powder

- ½ teaspoon sea salt

- 1 green chili, deseeded and chopped

- ½ teaspoon cinnamon

- 1 cup chopped yellow bell pepper

- ½ cup chopped red bell pepper

- 1 red onion, sliced

Procedure:

1. Heat the oil in a saucepan over medium-high flame. Add in onions and bell peppers and sauté for 5 minutes. Mix in the green chili, tomato puree, stevia, chili powder and cinnamon. Lower the heat and simmer the mixture for 15 minutes while stirring every 2 minutes.

2. While the mixture is simmering, place the paprika, salt, pepper and oregano in a large bowl and mix them together. Add the steak halves into the bowl and rub the spices all over it.

3. Place a non-stick grill pan on the stovetop with medium-high flame. Grill each side of the steak for 6 minutes, then let it cool down for 5 minutes. Once the steak is warm, slice it into long strips and arrange them on a serving plate.

4. Once the vegetables are tender and the sauce has thickened, pour the contents of the saucepan over the grilled steak slices and serve immediately.

Grilled Mustard Lamb Chops with Herbs

Tangy mustard mixed together with herbes de Provence creates an aromatic lamb chop marinade that will awaken the taste buds.

Serves: 4

Ready in: 20 minutes

Ingredients:

- 8 lamb chops

- 2 tablespoons Dijon mustard

- 1 teaspoon garlic powder

- 1 tablespoon dried herbes de Provence

- ½ teaspoon paprika

- ½ teaspoon salt

- 1 tablespoon olive oil

Procedure:

1. In a large bowl, mix together the mustard, garlic powder, paprika, salt and herbes de Provence. Add in the lamb chops and rub the spice mixture on both sides.

2. Heat half of the olive oil in a grill pan over medium-high flame. Place 4 lamb chops on the grill pan and cook each side for 4 minutes. Use the remaining olive oil to grill 4 more lamb chops at 4 minutes per side. Serve immediately.

Baked Pork Tenderloin

Pork tenderloin is a great choice meat for weight loss advocates because it is lean, juicy and quickly absorbs the zesty flavors of its marinade.

Serves: 4

Ready in: 40 minutes

Ingredients:

- 450 grams pork tenderloin
- 1 teaspoon olive oil
- 2 drops liquid stevia
- 2 teaspoons paprika
- ½ teaspoon onion powder
- 1 teaspoon garlic powder
- ½ teaspoon salt
- 1 teaspoon ground coffee granules
- ½ teaspoon ground black pepper
- ½ cup water
- 1 teaspoon grass-fed butter

Procedure:

1. Preheat the oven to 425°F and prepare an ovenproof skillet.

2. In a bowl, combine together paprika, salt, pepper, garlic powder, onion powder, stevia and coffee granules. Add in the pork and rub the mixture all over it.

3. Place the skillet on a stovetop with medium-high flame. Add the butter then the pork tenderloin and sear the sides until it becomes light brown. Transfer the skillet into the oven and bake for 15 minutes.

4. After 15 minutes, remove the skillet from the oven and transfer the pork to a chopping board. Let it stand for 5 minutes then slice into 1-inch cuts. Place the pork slices on a serving platter.

5. Pour water into the skillet and mix it with the drippings. Pour the sauce over the pork slices and serve immediately.

Asian Beef Stir-Fry

Wheat Belly dining has never tasted so delicious with this oriental-inspired dish that uses wheat-free condiments to add flavor to the beef.

Serves: 3

Ready in: 1 hour

Ingredients:

- 900 grams sirloin steak, cut into 2-inch strips
- 1 tablespoon olive oil
- 1 teaspoon crushed garlic
- 3 cups sliced shiitake mushrooms
- 1 Bok Choy, trimmed and chopped
- 1 drop liquid stevia
- 4 tablespoons coconut aminos
- 1 teaspoon minced ginger
- 1 ½ teaspoon ground flaxseeds
- ½ teaspoon ground black pepper
- 2 ½ tablespoons arrowroot powder

Procedure:

1   Blend together sirloin strips, pepper, ½ tablespoon arrowroot powder and 2 tablespoons coconut aminos in a mixing bowl. Cover with plastic wrap and leave it to marinade for 30 minutes.

2. In a separate bowl, mix together the remaining coconut aminos, arrowroot powder, stevia and ginger then set aside. This will serve as the sauce of the dish.

3. Heat the olive oil in a pan over medium-high heat. Cook the sirloin strips for 2 minutes per side then transfer to a plate. Once all the beef strips have been cooked and set aside, start sautéing the mushrooms, garlic and Bok Choy. Cook the vegetables for 2 minutes then return the meat back into the pan. Pour in the prepared sauce and cook the dish for 3 minutes. Serve while hot.

Pan-fried Pork Chops with Spiced Peaches

Stone fruits such as peaches, nectarines and plums are natural flavor enhancers that you can use to create delectable pork dishes.

Serves: 5

Ready in: 30 minutes

Ingredients:

- 5 bone-in pork chops
- 2 peaches, pitted and quartered
- 2 ½ tablespoons olive oil
- ¼ cup chopped mint leaves
- 1 white onion, quartered
- 2 tablespoons lemon juice
- 2 teaspoons Dijon mustard
- Pinch of sea salt and ground black pepper

Procedure:

1. Combine the peaches, onions, salt, pepper and 2 tablespoons olive oil in a saucepan and simmer over medium flame for 8

minutes or until the peaches are soft. Remove the saucepan from the heat and take out the peaches and onions.

2. Slice the peaches and onions into smaller chunks and return them to the saucepan. Mix the lemon juice, mint leaves and mustard into the peach sauce and set aside.

3. Heat the remaining olive oil in a large pan over medium-high heat. Place pork chops in the pan and cook each side for 3 minutes. Once the pork chops are cooked, pour in the peach sauce and simmer for 1 minute. Turn off the heat and serve while hot.

Chapter 7: Wheat Belly Chicken & Poultry Recipes

Parmesan Chicken Bites

The kids will love these homemade chicken nuggets that are peppered with Parmesan and flaxseeds for that extra crunch.

Serves: 4

Ready in: 30 minutes

Ingredients:

- ½ cup ground flaxseeds

- 2 eggs

- ½ cup shredded Parmesan cheese

- ¼ teaspoon garlic powder

- ¼ teaspoon sea salt

- ¼ teaspoon onion powder

- ¼ teaspoon ground black pepper

- 2 tablespoons grass-fed butter

- 450 grams boneless and skinless chicken breast, cubed

Procedure:

1. Preheat the oven to 350°F and prepare a parchment-lined baking sheet.

2. Combine the butter and egg in a small bowl and whisk them together. Set this aside.

3. In another bowl, mix together garlic powder, salt, pepper, flaxseeds, onion powder and cheese.

4. Dip each chicken piece into the egg mixture then dredge it in the flaxseed and cheese mixture to coat. Place the nuggets on the baking sheet and bake for 20 minutes. Serve while hot.

Gluten Free Baked Thyme Chicken

Apart from bringing out the lovely flavors of poultry, thyme also contains antiseptic properties that help fight fungi, coughs and skin infections.

Serves: 2

Ready in: 40 minutes

Ingredients:

- 2 boneless and skinless chicken breasts
- ½ cup homemade chicken stock
- 3 sprigs fresh thyme
- 5 garlic cloves, crushed
- 1 teaspoon lemon zest
- 1 tablespoon lemon juice
- Pinch of salt and ground black pepper
- Lemon wedges

Procedure:

1. Preheat the oven to 375°F and prepare a small baking dish.

2. Season the chicken breasts with salt and pepper then lay these inside the baking dish. Add in the garlic, thyme and lemon zest and rub it onto the chicken. Finally, pour the lemon juice and chicken stock into the baking dish and place it inside the oven.

3. Bake the chicken dish for 35-40 minutes while basting it with the sauce every 15 minutes. Serve the chicken breasts with a few lemon wedges on the side.

Fiery Sweet Chicken Thighs

Serve this mouth-watering chicken entrée that's coated with the wonderful flavors of stevia, salt and 7 fiery spices.

Serves: 4

Ready in: 45 minutes

Ingredients:

- 4 chicken thighs
- 1 teaspoon liquid stevia
- 2 teaspoons salt
- 2 tablespoons chili powder
- 2 teaspoons ground black pepper
- 1 teaspoon cayenne pepper
- 2 teaspoons mustard powder
- 2 teaspoons cumin
- 2 teaspoons paprika
- 2 tablespoons garlic powder

Procedure:

1. Place the chicken thighs in a bowl and rub the stevia around the meat and skin. Set this aside.

2. In a separate bowl, blend together the chili powder, black pepper, cayenne pepper, mustard powder, cumin, paprika and garlic powder. Dredge the chicken thighs into the bowl of spices, making sure to rub the spices on all corners of the meat.

3. Place a grill pan over medium-high flame and grease it with cooking spray. Once the grill is hot, place the chicken thighs on the pan with skin side down. Grill the chicken for 10-12 minutes, flip it, and grill for another 10 minutes.

4. Remove the chicken thighs from the grill and let it cool at room temperature for 10 minutes. Transfer the chicken to a plate and serve immediately.

Spicy Chicken and Tomato Skewers

This African-inspired chicken kebab dish will taste better when it's soaked in the spicy vinegar marinade overnight.

Serves: 6

Ready in: 1 hour

Ingredients:

- 900 grams boneless chicken breast, cut into 1½-inch chunks
- 12 cherry tomatoes
- 3 teaspoons chili powder
- ½ cup white vinegar
- 2 teaspoons paprika
- ¾ cup lemon juice
- 1 teaspoon oregano
- ¼ cup olive oil
- ½ teaspoon salt
- 2 garlic cloves, crushed
- 1 shallot, minced

Procedure:

1. Mix together the chili powder, olive oil, paprika, oregano, salt, garlic, shallots, vinegar and lemon juice in a large bowl. Add the chicken chunks into the spiced vinegar marinade and leave it soaking for 30 minutes or overnight.

2. While the chicken is marinating, soak the bamboo skewers in water for 5 minutes. Once the chicken is ready, get a cherry tomato and skewer it through the stick. Next, skewer 4-5 chicken chunks then end with another cherry tomato. Do the same process to make another 5 chicken kebabs.

3. Heat the grill pan over medium-high flame. Once the pan is hot, place the chicken skewers on the pan and cook for 10-12 minutes while turning every 2 minutes. Cook the kebabs until golden brown.

Wheat-Free Turkey Burgers with Lemon Dip

If you are craving for a quick snack after a morning workout, have a serving or two of this guilt-free turkey burger that won't pack on the pounds.

Makes: 10 patties

Ready in: 20 minutes

Ingredients:

- 450 grams ground turkey breast

- 1 egg, beaten

- 3 tablespoons chopped fresh parsley

- 2 green onions, chopped

- 1 zucchini, peeled and grated

- 1 garlic clove, minced

- ½ teaspoon cayenne pepper

- ½ teaspoon white pepper

- ½ teaspoon garlic powder

- 1 teaspoon salt

- ½ teaspoon cumin

- 2 teaspoons lemon juice

- 1 cup Greek yoghurt

- 2 tablespoons olive oil

- Pinch of sea salt

Procedure:

1. To make the creamy lemon dip, whisk together lemon juice, salt, yoghurt and 1 tablespoon olive oil. Set the dip aside.

2. In a separate bowl, mix together the ground turkey, egg, zucchini, green onions, garlic and the rest of the spices. Roll out 10 balls from the mixture then flatten it to make burger patties.

3. Heat the remaining oil in a large pan over medium-high flame. Once the oil is hot, cook the patties for 7 minutes or until golden brown. Flip the burgers then cook the other side for another 7 minutes.

4. Arrange the turkey burgers on a plate and serve it with the prepared dip.

Chapter 8: Wheat Belly Dessert Recipes

Wheat Belly Chocolate Chip Cookies

Stevia, a natural plant-based sweetener, was used to make this sweet yet healthy after-meal treat.

Makes: 25 cookies

Ready in: 40 minutes

Ingredients:

- 4 eggs
- 4 cups almond flour
- ½ teaspoon stevia extract
- 1 teaspoons vanilla extract
- 1 cup unsweetened dark chocolate chips
- ½ teaspoon salt
- ½ cup butter
- 1 teaspoon baking soda
- ¼ cup coconut milk

Procedure:

1. Line a cookie sheet with parchment and preheat the oven to 325°F.

2. Mix together the almond flour, salt and baking soda in a large bowl and set this aside.

3. In a separate bowl, mix together the eggs, stevia, coconut milk, butter and vanilla. Blend in the almond flour mixture and mix well. Fold in the chocolate chips and mix.

4. Drop tablespoons of the cookie dough onto the lined cookie sheet, making sure to press the cookie down to flatten it. Place the cookies in the oven and bake for 30 minutes. Once the cookies are ready, place these on an oven rack to cool.

Minty Avocado Cups

Revel over the beautiful layers of avocado, blueberry and ricotta in this gluten free dessert recipe.

Serves: 4

Ready in: 30 minutes

Ingredients:

- 1 avocado, peeled, pitted and chopped

- 2 mint leaves, chopped

- 1 cup ricotta cheese

- 1 cup blueberries

- 1 teaspoon ginger powder

- 1 teaspoon liquid stevia

Procedure:

1 In a small bowl, mix together the blueberries, mint leaves and stevia. Set this aside.

2. Place the avocado, ricotta and ginger powder in a blender and process until smooth. Spoon a layer of the avocado mixture at the bottom of 4 cups or glasses, then follow it with a layer of

the blueberry and mint blend. Place another layer of the avocado followed by the last layer of blueberries. Top the dessert with mint leaves and refrigerate for 15 minutes. This dessert is best served cold.

Banana Walnut Brownies

This delectable brownie recipe takes only 15 minutes to bake and uses organic, waistline-friendly ingredients such as bananas and almond flour.

Makes: 12 brownies

Ready in: 25 minutes

Ingredients:

- 2 ripe bananas cut into ½ inch thick slices
- ½ cup almond flour
- 2 teaspoons liquid stevia
- ¼ cup cocoa powder
- 2 tablespoons coconut milk
- 3 eggs
- 4 tablespoons organic butter, melted
- 1 tablespoon olive oil
- 1 teaspoon coconut oil
- ¼ teaspoon baking soda
- ½ teaspoon sea salt

- ½ cup chopped walnuts

Procedure:

1. Preheat the oven to 350°F and grease a 9 x 9 baking pan.

2. Place a grill pan over medium-high flame and heat the coconut oil. Place the pieces of banana on the pan and lightly brown each side. Once the bananas are golden brown, remove the pan from the heat.

3. In a large bowl, whisk together the eggs, coconut milk and butter. Add in the olive oil, baking soda, almond flour, stevia and cocoa powder. Mix the batter well then pour into the baking pan. Arrange the fried bananas and walnuts at the top of the brownie batter then place it inside the oven. Bake this for 15 minutes. Let the brownies cool for 10 minutes before slicing into equal portion.

Strawberry Apple Sherbet

A healthy serving of this cold dessert contains vitamins, natural sugars and healthy fats that will not disrupt weight loss efforts.

Serves: 6

Ready in: 5 hours 10 minutes

Ingredients:

- 1 cup coconut milk
- 2 cups sliced strawberries
- 2 apples, peeled, cored and sliced thinly
- 2 ripe bananas, peeled and mashed
- 1 tablespoon liquid stevia

Procedure:

1. Place the strawberries, bananas and apples in a blender and pulse until smooth. Pour in the stevia and coconut milk and blend it until the consistency becomes creamy.

2. Pour the sherbet mixture in a metal container and place it in the coldest part of the freezer for at least 5 hours. Once the mixture is frozen, scoop the sherbet into individual glasses and serve.

Spiced Fresh Fruit Plate

A sprinkle of cayenne pepper helps balance out the sweetness of fresh fruits. Moreover, this spice helps boost metabolism and controls appetite.

Serves: 6

Ready in: 15 minutes

Ingredients:

- 1 teaspoon cayenne pepper
- 2 drops liquid stevia
- 2 cups strawberries, trimmed and halved
- 2 peaches, pitted and chopped
- 1 red grapefruit, peeled and sectioned
- 2 kiwis, peeled and sliced
- 1 cup blueberries
- 1 mango, peeled, pitted and chopped
- 2 teaspoons lemon juice
- 1 tablespoon hot water
- 1 cup walnuts

Procedure:

1. In a small bowl, mix together the walnuts, stevia, hot water and cayenne pepper. Place the coated nuts on a baking sheet and broil it for 3 minutes, making sure that it does not burn.

2. Place the strawberries, blueberries, kiwis, peaches, mangoes, grapefruit and lemon juice in a bowl. Add in the spiced walnuts and toss. Serve in individual bowls.

Peach and Strawberry Bites

This freezer-friendly dessert tastes decadent, but is actually low in calories. Use dark semi-sweet chocolate chips that contain monounsaturated fatty acids that are proven to control cravings.

Servings: 4

Ready in: 25 minutes

Ingredients:

- 8 strawberries, trimmed and washed

- ½ cup dark chocolate chips, melted

- 1 peach, pitted and pureed

Procedure:

1. Core the strawberries with a small knife.

2. Place the peach puree in a small Ziploc bag and cut the corner to make a piping bag. Pipe the pureed fruit into the strawberries.

3. Place the strawberries on a plate then drizzle the melted chocolate on top of the dessert. Place the berries in the freezer. Serve these frozen.

Chapter 9: Easy Tips to Help You Cope with Wheat Withdrawal

"Once wheat-free, always wheat-free is the best policy."

Dr. William Davis

A major reason why some people who follow the Wheat Belly program slip back into old habits of eating processed food and sugars is the feeling of weakness, discomfort and mental anguish that is commonly present when beginning a gluten-free journey. If you have just transitioned to a wheat-free lifestyle yet feel symptoms such as nausea, depression, stomach trouble and joint pains, do not turn to junk food for comfort. Yours is a simple case of wheat withdrawal.

Two factors can cause wheat withdrawal: the sudden absence of gluten in the system and delayed oxidation of fat as a result of lesser calories. These changes may affect our minds and bodies at the start of a wheat-free program, but it becomes manageable as days pass. Before you know it, your body has become accustomed to a wheat-free diet that provides long-term health benefits.

To help you cope with the uncomfortable symptoms of wheat withdrawal, here are 5 simple tips that will keep you on the road towards reaching your goal weight:

1. Drink lots of water

   Going wheat-free reduces inflammation and water retention that are some of the known causes of weight gain. To help cope with fluid loss, drink at least 8 glasses of water a day or consume fruit-infused drinks that have zero sugar. This will regulate organ function and help curb appetite.

2. Take iodine supplements

   Iodine plays a huge role in weight loss as it regulates the hormones that sustain metabolic activity. Unfortunately, once a person stops consuming salty foods such as processed meat, iodine levels drop and he/she becomes weak and more likely to have heart, weight and cholesterol problems because of iodine deficiency. Take supplements that provide the body with at least 500mcg of iodine per day.

3. Boost your diet with omega-3 fatty acids

   Cutting wheat, sugars and processed foods from your diet leads to rapid weight loss, which in turn causes a voluminous release of fatty acids into the bloodstream. This activity causes high triglyceride levels. To help control your cholesterol, boost your omega-3 intake by taking fish oil capsules or eating foods such as fish, eggs and nuts. Omega 3 controls fatty acid mobilization by triggering enzymes that remove them from the bloodstream.

4. Consume probiotics

   Probiotic capsules and drinks help protect stomach health by introducing gut-friendly bacteria into the system. Hence, if you are experiencing diarrhea, constipation or any other stomach discomfort within 48 hours of removing gluten from your diet, take a probiotic supplement to help regulate bowel movement.

5. Always add salt to your meals

   Healthy salt such as sea salt can add flavor to dishes, provided you use it sparingly. Apart from making your Wheat Belly meals satisfying to the taste buds, salt helps prevent rapid fluid loss and over-fatigue. A pinch of salt added to a wheat-free entrée makes all the difference.

Wheat withdrawal is a common struggle for novice Wheat Belly practitioners. However, do not let these setbacks discourage you. Once you start seeing the amazing effects of going grain-free, you will realize that the changes, restrictions and efforts were all worth it.

Chapter 10: The Science behind a Gluten Free Diet

"It's bizarre that the produce manager is more important to my children's health then the pediatrician."

Meryl Streep

Over 20 million people across the world have adopted a zero-gluten lifestyle and have drastically changed the way they eat. Health food advocates have strongly claimed that eliminating wheat and other gluten-enriched products from their diet have helped them achieve a healthier body, clearer mind and a happier soul.

Let us find out the science behind this controversial protein and how it affects the balance within the human body:

The Composition of Gluten

Gluten in its simplest form is a protein found in food products made with wheat, barley, rye and other grain varieties. It is composed of two proteins: glutenin and gliadin. The reason why gluten grains are used in food preparation is due to its chemical composition that provides food with elasticity, thus making it softer and easier to chew.

It has been proven that bread has a high gluten content compared to most foods because the kneading process extracts more gluten strands and creates links with other proteins. However, processed food and artificial flavor enhancers have likewise been found to contain gluten, apart from other chemicals that are harmful to the body.

How Is Gluten Harmful to the Body?

A high consumption of gluten-enriched foods creates a negative autoimmune reaction within the body, hence making an individual more prone to allergies, illness and disorders. This response can be attributed to the body's reaction to gliadin, a sub-protein of gluten that creates abnormal activities within the digestive tract.

Once gluten enters the body and sticks to the digestive wall, the immune system treats it as a harmful element that needs to be eliminated. Automatically, the immune system attacks the gluten and in the process, damages the healthy cells of the stomach. The damaged cells of the intestines become the entry point for bacteria and other harmful chemicals into the body.

Some diseases that have been linked to regular gluten intake include celiac disease, irritable bowel syndrome, leaky gut syndrome, anemia, fatigue, food allergies and brain damage. Though celiac disease is known to be a genetically-inherited disease, other illnesses have developed due to gluten intolerance caused by eating huge portions of grain products.

The Benefits of a Gluten Free Diet

People who have taken the turn for the better and eliminated gluten from their diet have experienced the wonders of clean, healthy eating. Removing wheat products from one's diet and replacing it with fruits, vegetables, dairy and lean meats will help cleanse the system and protect the cells from degeneration.

Here are some of the health benefits of a gluten free diet:

- easier weight management

- less cravings for unhealthy food

- food allergies are eliminated

- treatment of celiac disease and other autoimmune diseases

- reduced IBS symptoms

- lesser risk of having stomach problems

- lower cholesterol and blood sugar levels

- reduced risk of heart disease and cancer

- have more energy for weight loss activities

- happier disposition

- brain disorder symptoms for people with autism, epilepsy and schizophrenia are easier to manage

Gluten Free Food Checklist

Before starting on your journey towards a healthier gluten free lifestyle, it is important to know which foods should be a part of your ingredient list and which ones should be eliminated from the pantry. Here is a list of foods to guide you in preparing healthier meals:

Safe Gluten Free Foods

- Gluten free flours and grains such as almond flour, millet, amaranth, buckwheat, sorghum, corn flour, cornmeal, potato flour, quinoa, rice (brown, white), teff flour, gluten free oats

- Fresh fruits, vegetables and herbs

- Beans, legumes and soy

- Healthy nuts and seeds

- Canned fruits, vegetables and juices, provided they do not contain artificial sweeteners or additives

- Dairy products such as butter, milk, eggs, cream, real cheese, gluten free yoghurt

- Red meat, chicken and seafood, provided that they are not breaded nor soaked in gluten-enriched marinades

- Healthy oils such as olive oil, coconut oil, sesame oil, canola oil

- Sweeteners such as sugar, honey, maple syrup, coconut sugar, agave

- Spices and seasonings such as vinegar, gluten free soy sauce, coconut aminos, ground spices, dried herbs

- Alcoholic beverages

- Baking products such as powdered pectin, xantham and guar gums, tapioca, baking powder, baking soda, vanilla

Gluten Products to Avoid

- Wheat-enriched recipes made with wheat flour, couscous, semolina, kamut, spelt, durum, triticale, modified wheat starch, cake flour

- Malt products such as malt vinegar, malt syrup, malt flavoring

- Barley products such as licorice, mock seafood meat, beer

- Artificial seasonings, sauces and marinades

- Rye

- Processed cheeses and cheese spreads

- Breads and pastries such as cakes, doughnuts, muffins, pretzels

In order to create a healthier kitchen, always check the grocery for gluten free alternatives of your favorite food. Otherwise, it is always best to stick to using organic, wheat-free ingredients when preparing meals for you and the whole family.

Transitioning to a gluten free lifestyle may seem challenging at first, but its benefits are worth every simple change that you are willing to make to your daily eating habits. Dining healthy and gluten free will help you achieve total wellness and a better life ahead.

Gluten free dishes can be prepared in a number of ways: grilling, frying, baking or steaming. However, an easier way to cook these delicious recipes is by using a slow cooker. You get the same flavor and nutrition without the hassle of spending countless hours in the kitchen.

The succeeding chapter will discuss the benefits of having a slow cooker in your gluten free kitchen and a few tips on how it can help novice chefs prepare nutritious and tasty meals.

Chapter 11: Slow Cooker Tips for Gluten Free Dishes

If you are a greenhorn at the kitchen, chances are you already feel intimidated by the thought of cutting, dicing, frying, baking, boiling and plating dishes for a lengthy amount of time. Let's face it: cooking delicious and gluten free treats does require a lot of time and energy.

However, there is a way to unburden your culinary anxiety, and that is by using a reliable and efficient slow cooker. It will simplify the cooking process and allow you to relax and enjoy your time while a delicious home-cooked meal is being prepared.

A slow cooker is every beginner chef's dream machine. Apart from it costing cheaper than an oven or outside grill, creating meals in a slow cooker is quick and easy. Just prepare the ingredients, place them all inside the pot, cover it, set the time and temperature then wait for the dish to cook. After a few hours, your gluten free recipe will turn out as appetizing as any other stove-top meal could be.

On the other hand, there is a huge difference between slow-cooking your ingredients and cooking great slow cooker dishes. Here are 6 basic tips that will help you create mouth-watering gluten free food while utilizing the incredible features of a slow cooker:

- Consider the right size slow cooker for your kitchen needs

  If you are planning on purchasing a slow cooker, think of the volume of cooking that you usually do. If you have a small family of four, a 5-quart slow cooker would suit your kitchen. On the other hand, if you live solo and want to cook simple, gluten free meals while you are away at work, a smaller 3 ½ quart slow cooker will do.

The right size pot will enable you to cook ingredients properly without spilling over once the dish starts to simmer.

- Determine the most suitable cooking time and temperature

The slow cooker recipes in this book are flexible in terms of cooking time and can be set on either low or high temperatures. However, it would be best to determine the most suitable range for each dish as this would affect its quality and flavor.

Here is a basic measure of temperature and cooking time if you choose to prepare food in a slow cooker:

- If the recipe calls for a cooking time of less than 30 minutes, slow cook the dish on high heat for 2 hours or cook it on low heat for 6 hours;

- If the recipe calls for a cooking time of 30 minutes to an hour, slow cook the dish on high heat for 3 hours or cook it on low heat for 7 hours;

- If the recipe calls for a cooking time of 1-2 hours, slow cook the dish on high heat for 4 hours or cook it on low heat for 8 hours; and

- If the recipe calls for a cooking time of 2-4 hours, slow cook the dish on high heat for 5 hours or cook it on low heat for 9 hours.

For example, if you are preparing for dinner in the late afternoon, it is suggested that you cook your dish on high heat so that the process is quicker and the meal will be done in 3-4 hours.

On the other hand, it is advisable to cook gluten free dishes on low heat if you have enough time. This method may add another 3 hours of cooking but the lengthy simmering of ingredients will bring out the flavors of the dish.

- Keep the pot covered

Once you have set the time and the temperature of the slow cooker, cover it and leave it as it is unless the recipe requires you to mix the dish often. Frequent uncovering of the lid will release the heat inside the pot and affect the quality of your dish. This will likewise lead to adjustments in the timer and dishes take longer to cook than expected.

Prepare your dishes in advance

Slow cookers are great kitchen appliances that will help you prepare flavorful meals for the family. In this light, it does help that a little planning and preparation is involved so that you can leave your slow cooker in the morning and allow the dish to be cooked while you are doing your daily activities.

Plan your slow cooker meals the night before. Slice and prepare the ingredients, place them in containers and chill them overnight. In the morning, mix all your ingredients in the slow cooker and leave it there to cook for hours. Experience the wonders of cooking without being stuck inside the kitchen.

• Brown your meat and onions for a little extra flavor

An extra tip to make gluten free meals more flavorful: if you have extra time on your hands, brown your onions and meat in a skillet before cooking it in a slow cooker. When you sauté your ingredients beforehand, the meat and onions caramelize and a savory glaze sticks to it. This adds a bit of sweetness and smokiness to the dish.

• Be experimental when preparing dishes in a slow cooker

This part contains 40 gluten free recipes that can be prepared with the ease of a slow cooker. Use the slow cooker to prepare breakfast, sauces, main entrées and even desserts: the possibilities are limitless. Be creative while cooking gluten free recipes. You will subsequently realize that owning a slow cooker gives you the freedom to enjoy quality time while concocting healthy and scrumptious meals for the whole family.

Gluten free dishes will be taste much better with these basic slow cooker tips. Try them out for yourself and make slow cooking a part of your healthy daily habits.

Chapter 12: Delicious and Gluten Free Breakfast Recipes

Slow Cooker Potato and Sausage Casserole

Preparation time: 30 minutes

Cooking time: 5 hours

Number of servings: 4

Ingredients:

- 1 ½ cups shredded potatoes

- 6 eggs, beaten

- 1 cup lean ground sausage

- ½ cup shredded Parmesan cheese

- 2 garlic cloves, minced

- ½ yellow onion, sliced

- ¼ cup fresh milk

- ½ tablespoon Dijon mustard

- Pinch of salt and pepper

Directions:

1. Lightly grease the inside of the slow cooker with oil spray. Lay down the shredded potatoes inside the pot.

2. In a small bowl, mix together the beaten eggs, milk, mustard, salt and pepper. Set this aside.

3. Place a frying pan over medium high heat and sauté the garlic, onions and sausage. Once the sausage has turned golden brown, remove it from the heat and drain the excess oil. Place the browned sausage meat mixture on top of the grated potatoes.

4. Sprinkle the grated cheese on top of the sausage meat. Slowly pour in the egg mixture over the sausage and potato layers and mix them together so that the ingredients are evenly distributed.

5. Cover the pot and adjust the temperature to high. Cook the casserole for 5 hours until the casserole is firm to the touch.

6. Place the casserole in a serving plate and enjoy!

Cinnamon Apple Oatmeal

Preparation time: 15 minutes

Cooking Time: 7 hours

Number of servings: 2

Ingredients:

- 2 cups peeled and chopped red apples

- 2 cups gluten free oatmeal

- 1 teaspoon cinnamon powder

- 2 tablespoons coconut oil

- ½ cup coconut sugar

- ½ cup fresh milk

Directions:

1. Place the chopped apples in a slow cooker.

2. Add the cinnamon powder, coconut oil and coconut sugar to the apples and mix well.

3. Cover the pot and set the temperature to low. Slow-cook the oatmeal overnight for at least 7 hours.

4. Spoon the oatmeal into individual bowls and drizzle some milk on top before serving.

Breakfast Rice Pudding

Preparation time: 5 minutes

Cooking time: 2 hours

Number of servings: 4

Ingredients:

- ¾ cup short grain white rice
- 1 cup water
- 1 ½ cup evaporated milk
- ½ cup honey
- ½ cup golden raisins
- ½ teaspoon cinnamon
- ½ teaspoon vanilla
- ½ teaspoon salt

Directions:

1. Place the rice, water milk, honey, raisins, cinnamon, vanilla and salt in a slow cooker and mix well.

2. Cover the slow cooker and set the temperature to high. Cook the pudding for 2 hours and stir every 30 minutes.

3. Divide the pudding into individual bowls and serve it warm.

Slow Cooker Apple Spread on Toast

Preparation time: 15 minutes

Cooking time: 9 hours

Number of servings: 8

Ingredients:

- 12 Fuji apples, peeled and cored
- 2 teaspoons cinnamon powder
- 2 cups coconut sugar
- ¼ teaspoon salt
- ¼ teaspoon cloves
- 8 slices gluten-free bread, toasted

Directions:

1. Chop the apples and place them in a slow cooker.

2. Add in the cinnamon powder, coconut sugar, salt and cloves to the pot and mix well.

3. Cover the slow cooker and set the temperature to high. Cook the apples for an hour but stir the mixture every 15 minutes.

4. After an hour, adjust the slow cooker temperature to low and continue cooking the apple spread for 8 more hours.

5. Once the apple spread is done, remove the lid and let it cool down to room temperature. Pour the spread into a bowl or jar

then serve the apple spread with toasted gluten free bread for breakfast.

Cheese and Spinach Frittata

Preparation time: 10 minutes

Cooking time: 1 hour 30 minutes

Number of servings: 4

Ingredients:

- 1 ½ cups chopped spinach leaves

- 1 cup cottage cheese

- ½ cup chopped yellow onion

- 1 tomato, diced

- 3 tablespoons fresh milk

- 2 eggs

- 2 egg whites

- Salt and pepper to taste

Directions:

1. Lightly brown the onions on a skillet and set this aside.

2. Whisk the eggs and egg whites in a bowl. Add in the spinach, cheese, tomato, fresh milk, salt and pepper and mix well.

3. Pour the frittata mixture into a slow cooker, cover it and set the temperature to low.

4. Cook the frittata for 1 ½ hours until the eggs have been fully cooked.

5. Transfer the frittata to a plate before serving.

Banana Quinoa Cereal

Preparation time: 10 minutes

Cooking time: 5 hours

Number of servings: 6

Ingredients:

- 1 ½ cups quinoa

- 2 bananas, mashed

- 4 tablespoons honey

- 1 tablespoon light cream

- 1 cup fresh milk

- 1 cup water

- ½ teaspoon vanilla extract

- 2 tablespoons melted butter

- 2 tablespoons chopped almonds

- Banana slices

Directions:

1. Mix the honey and almonds in a bowl and blend well.

2. Place the quinoa, light cream, fresh milk, water, vanilla and melted butter in a slow cooker. Add in the mashed bananas and the honey and nut mixture. Mix the ingredients well.

3. Cover the pot and cook the cereal on low for 5 hours.

4. Once the cereal is done, mix it with a wooden spoon and pour it into a serving bowl. Place a few slices of banana on top to garnish the cereal.

Slow Cooker Hard-boiled Eggs

Preparation time: 5 minutes

Cooking time: 8 hours

Number of servings: 8

Ingredients:

- 8 medium eggs

- 3 cups water

- 1 tablespoon olive oil

- 2 tablespoons ground coffee

Directions:

1. Place the eggs, olive oil and ground coffee in a slow cooker.

2. Set the temperature to the lowest range and cover the pot. Simmer the eggs for 8 hours.

3. Peel the hard-boiled eggs before serving.

Homemade Strawberry Jam

Preparation time: 20 minutes

Cooking time: 4 hours

Number of servings: 5

Ingredients:

- 8 cups fresh strawberries, rinsed and hulled
- 3 cups granulated sugar
- 3 tablespoons fresh orange juice
- 4 tablespoons powdered pectin

Directions:

1. Place the strawberries in a large bowl and crush them with a potato masher or a hand blender. Once the berries are crushed, place them in a slow cooker.

2. Add the orange juice and powdered pectin to the crushed berries. Let it stand for 5-10 minutes.

3. Pour the sugar into the slow cooker and mix well. Cover the pot and set the temperature to low. Cook the berries for 2 hours while stirring every 30 minutes.

4. After 2 hours, remove the cover of the slow cooker and adjust the temperature to high. Cook the jam for another 2 hours.

5. Pour the jam into heat resistant jars and let them cool down. Spread the jam onto your favorite morning pancakes or waffles.

Chapter 13: Non-Gluten Soups and Stews Slow-Cooked to Perfection

Hearty Tomato Soup

Preparation time: 15 minutes

Cooking time: 6 hours

Number of servings: 6

Ingredients:

- 4 cups diced fresh tomatoes
- 4 cups natural chicken stock
- 2 celery stalks, diced
- 1 tablespoon chopped basil
- 2 carrots, peeled and diced
- 1 onion, chopped
- 1 cup heavy cream
- 2 teaspoons sea salt
- ½ cup grated Parmesan cheese

Directions:

1. Place the tomatoes, chicken broth, celery, carrots and onion inside the slow cooker. Cover the pot and cook the tomato mixture for 5 hours on high temperature.

2. Once the vegetables are tender, pour the contents of the slow cooker into a blender but do pass it through a strainer. Discard the remaining solids and puree the tomato mixture until it becomes smooth.

3. Pour the pureed tomato mixture back into the slow cooker then mix in the cream, salt and basil. Cover the pot and cook the soup for another hour.

4. Once the soup is ready, pour it into a serving bowl and top it with the grated Parmesan cheese.

Chicken Soup for the Gluten-free Soul

Preparation time: 20 minutes

Cooking time: 5 hours

Number of servings: 4

Ingredients:

- 4 chicken breasts, rinsed and dried
- 7 garlic cloves, minced
- 1 tablespoon olive oil
- 8 baby potatoes, sliced
- 2 zucchinis, peeled and diced
- 1 yellow bell pepper, deseeded and diced
- 1 yellow summer squash, peeled and diced
- 2 cups shredded cabbage
- 2 medium tomatoes, diced
- 1 teaspoon oregano
- 1 teaspoon dried basil
- 1 teaspoon chopped fresh parsley
- 3 cups natural chicken broth
- 1 teaspoon balsamic vinegar

- ½ teaspoon honey

- Salt and pepper to taste

Directions:

1. Drizzle the olive oil inside the crock pot then place the chicken breasts inside. Sprinkle some salt, pepper and the minced garlic on top of the chicken. Set this aside.

2. In a separate bowl, mix together the potatoes, zucchinis, tomatoes, bell pepper, summer squash, cabbage, oregano, basil and parsley. Toss the vegetables with the spices then add in the balsamic vinegar, honey and a sprinkle of salt and pepper.

3. Pour the mixed vegetables on top of the chicken breasts then add in the chicken broth.

4. Cover the pot then place the temperature on high. Cook the soup for 5 hours or until the chicken is very tender.

Spicy Eggplant Stew

Preparation time: 15 minutes

Cooking time: 8 hours

Number of servings: 8

Ingredients:

- ½ cup fresh vegetable stock
- 1 ½ cup pureed tomatoes
- 2 garlic cloves, minced
- 2 ½ cups diced eggplant
- 1 cup chopped red onion
- 1 ½ cups diced zucchini
- 1 large tomato, chopped
- 1 ½ cups diced butternut squash
- 1 medium carrot, peeled and julienned
- 3 pieces frozen okra
- ¼ teaspoon paprika
- ¼ teaspoon chili powder
- ½ teaspoon cumin powder
- ½ teaspoon turmeric powder

- ½ teaspoon ground black pepper

- ½ teaspoon salt

Directions:

1. Place the vegetable stock and pureed tomatoes inside the slow cooker. Add in the eggplant, garlic, onion, zucchini, tomato, butternut squash, carrot and okra and mix.

2. Add in all the spices into the stew and mix well. Cover the pot and set the temperature to low. Cook the stew for 8 hours or until the vegetables are soft. Pour the eggplant stew into a large soup bowl before serving.

Slow-cooked Chili con Carne

Preparation time: 15 minutes

Cooking time: 6 hours

Number of servings: 6

Ingredients:

- 450 grams ground beef
- 1 cup beef stock
- 1 teaspoon chili powder
- 1 teaspoon paprika
- 2 teaspoons cinnamon powder
- 1 red bell pepper, deseeded and diced
- 2 cups diced tomatoes
- 1 yellow onion, chopped
- 2 garlic cloves, minced
- 2 cups pureed pumpkin
- 1 cup diced green chilies

Directions:

1. Place the ground beef in the slow cooker and set the temperature to low.

2. Add in the beef stock, chili powder, paprika and cinnamon powder into the slow cooker and mix. Stir in the bell pepper, tomatoes, onion, garlic, pureed pumpkin and green chilies.

3. Cover the pot and cook the chili for 6 hours.

The Ultimate Sweet Potato Soup

Preparation time: 15 minutes

Cooking time: 8 hours

Number of servings: 8

Ingredients:

- 3 sweet potatoes, peeled and diced
- 1 cup chopped green beans
- 2 cups freshly-chopped tomatoes
- 1 yellow onion, chopped
- 3 celery stalks, chopped
- 1 ½ cup green lentils
- 4 carrots, chopped
- 5 garlic cloves, minced
- 8 cups natural broth (vegetable or chicken)
- 1 teaspoon dried oregano
- 1 teaspoon fresh rosemary
- Salt and pepper to taste

Directions:

1. Set the temperature of the slow cooker to low.

2. Add the sweet potatoes, green beans, tomatoes, onion, celery, lentils, carrots and garlic cloves into the slow cooker. Pour in the broth then sprinkle the oregano, rosemary, salt and pepper.

3. Cover the pot and cook the sweet potato soup for 8 hours. Add a little more broth in the end if the soup seems too thick.

Quinoa and Beans Stew

Preparation time: 20 minutes

Cooking time: 5 hours

Number of servings: 8

Ingredients:

- 450 grams dried black beans, rinsed
- 1 cup raw quinoa, rinsed
- 6 cups water
- 2 dried red chilies
- 3 ½ cups chopped tomatoes
- 3 garlic cloves, minced
- 1 red onion, chopped
- 2 green bell peppers, deseeded and chopped
- ½ cup chopped fresh cilantro
- 1 teaspoon coriander powder
- 2 ½ teaspoons chili powder
- 1 teaspoon cinnamon powder
- Salt and pepper to taste
- Handful of chopped green onions

Directions:

1. Place the black beans and quinoa into the slow cooker. Add in the water, chilies, tomatoes, garlic, onion, bell peppers and cilantro and stir.

2. Sprinkle the coriander, chili and cinnamon powders on top of the stew. Finally, season it with salt and pepper.

3. Cover the slow cooker and cook the stew on high for 5 hours. Sprinkle the chopped green onions on top before serving.

Slow Cooker Squash Soup

Preparation time: 15 minutes

Cooking time: 4 hours

Number of servings: 4

Ingredients:

- 2 cups chicken broth

- 1 cup fresh milk

- 2 cups chopped squash

- 2 teaspoons chopped cilantro

- 2 celery stalks, chopped

- ½ cup chopped carrots

- ¼ teaspoon salt

- ¼ teaspoon ground black pepper

- ½ cup grated Parmesan cheese

Directions:

1. Place the chicken broth, squash, celery, carrots, salt and pepper in a slow cooker and mix them well. Cover the pot and set the temperature to high. Cook the soup for 4 hours until the vegetables are very soft.

2. Uncover the pot and pour in the fresh milk. Mix the soup before pouring it in a serving bowl.

3. Sprinkle the cilantro and cheese on top of the soup before serving.

Warm and Chunky Corn Chowder

Preparation time: 10 minutes

Cooking time: 6 hours

Number of servings: 4

Ingredients:

- 8 cups natural chicken broth

- 2 cups fresh or frozen corn kernels

- 1 carrot, peeled and chopped

- 1 large potato, chopped

- 1 red onion, chopped

- 1 red bell pepper, deseeded and chopped

- 1 tablespoon olive oil

Directions:

1. Heat the olive oil in a pan and lightly sauté the onions.

2. Once the onions have slightly browned, place them inside the slow cooker and add in the corn, potato, carrot, onion and bell pepper. Mix them well.

3. Cover the slow cooker and set the temperature to high. Slow cook the chowder for 6 hours then turn it off.

4. Pour the chowder into a blender and pulse for 2-3 times, making sure to leave some vegetable chunks in the chowder. Place the mixture in soup bowls before serving.

Chapter 14: Delightfully Simple Gluten Free Main Dishes

Slow-cooked Sweet Ham

Preparation time: 5 minutes

Cooking time: 6 hours 30 minutes

Number of servings: 8

Ingredients:

- 3 kg bone-in ham, unwrapped
- 3 cups pineapple juice
- 1 cup maple syrup
- ½ cup brown sugar

Directions:

1. Place the ham in a large slow cooker. Rub the brown sugar on all sides of the meat.
2. Pour the pineapple juice and maple syrup on top of the ham.
3. Cover the pot and set the temperature to low. Cook for 7 hours or until the ham is tender once a fork is poked into it.
4. Turn off the slow cooker and let the ham stand for 20 minutes.

5. Remove the ham from the slow cooker and place it on a cutting board. Cut a few slices of the ham and place it on a serving dish together with the whole meat. Pour the sauce over the meat before serving.

Spicy Honey Sesame Chicken

Preparation time: 10 minutes

Cooking time: 4 hours

Number of servings: 6

Ingredients:

- 1 pound boneless and skinless chicken breasts
- 1 tablespoon chili powder
- 3 tablespoons raw honey
- 2 teaspoons sesame oil
- 2 tablespoons pureed tomatoes
- 1 teaspoon chopped chilies
- 1 teaspoon sesame seeds
- 1 teaspoon chopped green onions
- ½ cup chopped yellow onion
- 2 tablespoons apple cider vinegar
- 3 tablespoons gluten-free soy sauce
- 2 tablespoons water
- 1 teaspoon minced garlic
- 2 teaspoons corn starch

Directions:

1. Dissolve the corn starch in water until it is free of lumps. Set this aside.

2. In a separate bowl, mix together the soy sauce, apple cider vinegar, sesame oil, honey, chili powder and pureed tomatoes. Add in the yellow onions, garlic, chilies and chicken breasts and mix well.

3. Place the chicken breasts inside the slow cooker and pour the sauce on top. Cover the slow cooker and set the temperature to high. Cook for 4 hours or until the chicken is tender.

4. Top with green onions and sesame seeds before serving.

Slow-cooked Cabbage Rolls with Quinoa

Preparation time: 15 minutes

Cooking time: 6 hours

Number of servings: 8

Ingredients:

- 450 grams lean ground beef
- 8 cabbage leaves, boiled and drained
- ½ cup raw quinoa, washed and drained
- ¼ cup soy milk
- 2 garlic cloves, minced
- 1 red onion, minced
- 1 egg, beaten
- ¼ teaspoon ground black pepper
- ½ teaspoon salt
- 2 teaspoons gluten-free soy sauce
- 2 tablespoons coconut sugar
- 2 tablespoons apple cider vinegar
- 2 cups chopped tomatoes

Directions:

1. In a small bowl, combine the chopped tomatoes, apple cider vinegar, coconut sugar and soy sauce. Mix well and set aside.

2. On another bowl, mix together the ground beef, quinoa, soy milk, garlic, onion, egg, salt and pepper. Spoon a quarter cup of the beef mixture on the middle of a cabbage leaf, fold the sides over and roll it away from you. Do the same procedure for the rest of the cabbage leaves.

3. Place the cabbage rolls inside the slow cooker. Pour the tomato mixture inside the pot and cover it.

4. Set the temperature to low and cook the cabbage rolls for 6 hours. Place the rolls on a serving dish and pour the sauce over it before serving.

Lamb Curry with White Rice

Preparation time: 15 minutes

Cooking time: 3 hours

Number of servings: 3

Ingredients:

- 450 grams lamb shoulder
- 2 cups cooked white rice
- 1 ½ cup coconut milk
- 3 garlic cloves, minced
- 1 yellow onion, chopped
- 1 ½ tablespoons chopped ginger
- 2 tablespoons apple cider vinegar
- 1 teaspoon curry powder
- ¼ teaspoon turmeric powder
- ½ teaspoon mustard seeds
- ½ teaspoon ground coriander
- 1 teaspoon ground cumin
- ¼ teaspoon cinnamon powder

- ¼ teaspoon cayenne pepper

- 1 teaspoon salt

- ½ teaspoon ground black pepper

- ½ cup chopped fresh cilantro

Directions:

1. Prepare the lamb by cutting it at the bone. Set this aside.

2. Pour the coconut milk into the slow cooker. Add in the garlic, onion, ginger and vinegar and mix well.

3. Mix the curry powder, turmeric, mustard seeds, coriander, cumin, cinnamon, cayenne, salt and pepper into the coconut milk mixture.

4. Place the lamb pieces into the coconut milk and spices and mix well.

5. Cover the slow cooker and set the temperature on high. Cook the lamb curry for 3 hours, until the meat separates from the bone.

6. Once the meat is cooked, remove the bone pieces and discard.

7. Place the cooked white rice on a serving dish. Spoon the lamb curry and place it on top of the rice, and sprinkle fresh cilantro on top before serving.

Creamy Beef Stroganoff

Preparation time: 15 minutes

Cooking time: 4 hours

Number of servings: 6

Ingredients:

- 900 grams lean ground beef
- 1 tablespoon olive oil
- 2 cups button mushrooms, halved
- 2 yellow onions, chopped
- 1 tablespoon minced garlic
- 1 cup coconut milk
- 1 cup plain yoghurt
- 1 cup natural beef stock
- 2 tablespoons gluten free soy sauce
- 2 tablespoons non-gluten mustard
- Pinch of salt and pepper

Directions:

1. Heat the olive oil in a large skillet over medium heat. Fry the ground beef until it becomes slightly brown. Sprinkle some salt and pepper to taste. Once the beef is cooked, place it inside a large slow cooker.

2. Add the mushrooms, onions, garlic, mustard and soy sauce to the ground beef and mix well. Lastly, pour in the coconut milk and beef stock and cover the slow cooker.

3. Set the temperature to high and slow cook the beef for 3 ½ hours. Once the beef is cooked, pour it into a serving bowl and let it stand for 30 minutes. Spoon the yoghurt into the stroganoff and mix well before serving.

Gluten Free Vegan Gumbo

Preparation time: 20 minutes

Cooking time: 8 hours

Number of servings: 6 servings

Ingredients:

- 1 cup sliced okra
- 1 cup button mushrooms, halved
- 1 red onion, chopped
- 2 celery stalks, chopped
- 1 yellow bell pepper, deseeded and chopped
- 1 zucchini, sliced into quarters
- 1 eggplant, diced
- 3 garlic cloves, chopped
- 2 cups chopped tomatoes
- 2 cups canned kidney beans, washed and drained
- 2 cups water
- 3 tablespoons olive oil
- 2 tablespoons gluten free flour

- 2 tablespoons coconut aminos or non-gluten soy sauce

- 1 tablespoon chili powder

- ½ tablespoon cayenne pepper

- ½ tablespoon salt

- ½ tablespoon ground black pepper

- 3 cups cooked white rice

Directions:

1. In a large skillet over medium flame, heat a tablespoon of the olive oil. Start sautéing the okra, mushrooms, onion, celery, bell pepper, zucchini and eggplant until slightly brown. Place the sautéed vegetables inside the slow cooker.

2. On the same skillet, heat the remaining olive oil and add in the flour. Stir constantly while slowly pouring in the water. Allow the water to boil then pour it into the slow cooker.

3. Add the tomatoes, kidney beans, coconut aminos, chili powder, cayenne powder, salt and pepper into the slow cooker. Mix all the ingredients and place a lid on the slow cooker.

4. Adjust the cooker's temperature to low and cook the gumbo for 8 hours.

5. Place the cooked rice on a serving platter. Pour the cooked gumbo on top of the rice and serve immediately.

Slow-cooked Herb Chicken

Preparation time: 15 minutes

Cooking time: 6 hours

Number of servings: 4

Ingredients:

- 7 garlic cloves, minced
- 1 yellow onion, chopped
- 1 carrot, peeled and chopped
- ½ teaspoon sea salt
- ½ teaspoon whole pepper
- 1 teaspoon sage
- 2 teaspoons rosemary
- 1 teaspoon thyme
- 1 whole chicken, neck and insides removed
- 3 cups cooked white rice or quinoa

Directions:

1. Rinse the chicken with cold water and drain.
2. Place the chopped onions and carrots inside the chicken and the chopped garlic in between the skin and the meat.

3. In a small bowl, mix together the salt, pepper, sage, rosemary and thyme. Rub the spices onto the chicken.

4. Place the chicken inside the slow cooker and adjust the temperature to high. Cover the pot and roast the chicken for 6 hours until the meat falls off the bone.

5. Serve this dish with cooked rice or quinoa.

Slow Cooker Spicy Pork Chops

Preparation time: 20 minutes

Cooking time: 6 hours

Number of servings: 2

Ingredients:

- 4 pork chops
- 1 tablespoon gluten free soy sauce
- 1/3 cup water
- 1 tablespoon olive oil
- 1 cup gluten free ketchup (ex. Heinz)
- 1 teaspoon chili powder
- ½ cup chopped yellow onion
- 2 garlic cloves
- Pinch of salt and pepper

Directions:

1. Place a skillet over medium heat and heat the olive oil. Add the onions to the pan and sauté until it turn light brown.

2. Next, add in the garlic, ketchup, soy sauce, salt, pepper, chili powder and water. Allow the sauce to simmer for 8-10 minutes.

3. Place the pork chops inside the slow cooker and pour the sauce over it. Cover the pot and cook the pork chops on low heat for 6 hours.

4. Once the chops are cooked, place them on a serving dish and drizzle the sauce on top.

Chapter 15: Slow Cooker Dessert Recipes for the Sweet

Gluten Free Brownie Balls

Preparation time: 10 minutes

Cooking time: 3 hours

Number of servings: 8

Ingredients:

- 1 cup unsweetened cocoa powder
- 2 cups almond flour
- 2 eggs, beaten
- 1 cup coconut sugar
- ½ cup coconut milk
- ½ cup water
- ½ cup coconut oil
- 2 teaspoons baking soda
- 2 teaspoons baking powder
- 2 teaspoons vanilla
- 1 teaspoon salt

Directions:

1. Drizzle the coconut oil in the slow cooker and spread it around the base.

2. Place the flour, cocoa powder, sugar, baking powder, baking soda and salt into the pot and mix well.

3. Pour the eggs, coconut milk, water and vanilla onto the dry ingredients and blend them together with a wooden spoon.

4. Cover the pot and cook the brownie batter on low for 3 hours.

5. After 3 hours, turn off the slow cooker and let the brownie batter cool for 30 minutes. Once it has cooled down, scoop tablespoonfuls of the mixture then use your hands to form them into balls. Place them on a nice dish and serve.

Slow-cooked Bananas Foster

Preparation time: 15 minutes

Cooking time: 2 hours

Number of servings: 5

Ingredients:

- 5 bananas, peeled and sliced
- 1 cup coconut sugar
- 4 tablespoons melted butter
- ½ cup chopped almonds
- ¼ cup rum
- ½ teaspoon cinnamon powder
- ½ cup grated coconut

Directions:

1. In a small bowl, mix together the coconut sugar, butter, rum and cinnamon. Set this aside.

2. Arrange the banana slices inside the slow cooker. Pour the sugar and rum mixture on top of the bananas and cover it.

3. Cook the bananas on low heat for 2 hours. Sprinkle the coconut and almonds on top within the last 15 minutes of cooking.

4. Serve this dessert by itself or with a scoop of vanilla ice cream.

Scrumptious Crème Brulee

Preparation time: 10 minutes

Cooking time: 4 hours

Number of servings: 4

Ingredients:

- 5 egg yolks

- ½ cup white sugar

- ¼ cup raw sugar

- 2 cups whipping cream

- 1 tablespoon vanilla

Directions:

1. In a large bowl, whip the egg yolks while slowly adding the white sugar and whipping cream. Add in the vanilla and mix well.

2. Place the crème brulee mixture in a baking dish that will fit inside the slow cooker. Set this aside.

3. To create a water bath for the crème brulee, pour some water into the slow cooker. Place the baking dish with the crème brulee mixture inside of it while making sure that the water is halfway up the top of the baking dish.

4. Cover the slow cooker. Set the temperature to high and cook the crème brulee for 4 hours.

5. After 4 hours, turn off the slow cooker and remove the baking dish. Let the dessert cool for 30 minutes.

6. Sprinkle the raw sugar on top then slightly brown it with a handy butane torch to create a crisp topping. Serve immediately.

Slow Cooker Caramelized Peaches

Preparation time: 20 minutes

Cooking time: 2 hours

Number of servings: 10

Ingredients:

- 10 peaches, peeled, pitted and sliced
- ½ cup butter
- 1 cup coconut sugar
- ½ teaspoon powdered cloves
- ½ teaspoon cinnamon powder
- Scoop of gluten free ice cream*

Directions:

1. Place peaches, butter, coconut sugar, cloves and cinnamon in a slow cooker and mix.

2. Set the temperature to low and cover the slow cooker. Leave the peaches to caramelize for 2 hours then turn off the heat.

3. To arrange this dessert, divide the peaches into individual bowls and place a scoop of ice cream on top. Serve immediately.

4. Gluten free ice cream variants are available among popular brands such as Haagen-Dazs, Edy's and Breyer's. Be sure to check the labels.

Banana Bread Pudding

Preparation time: 15 minutes

Cooking time: 2 hours

Number of servings: 5

Ingredients:

- 5 bananas, peeled and chopped
- 6 cups cubed gluten free bread
- ½ cup maple syrup
- ½ cup granulated sugar
- ½ cup toasted pecans
- Pinch of salt
- 1 teaspoon brandy or rum
- ½ teaspoon minced ginger
- ½ teaspoon cinnamon powder
- ½ teaspoon nutmeg
- ½ cup almond milk
- 1 teaspoon butter

Directions:

1. In a mixing bowl, combine the sugar, pecans, brandy and bananas. Mix them well and set it aside.

2. In a separate bowl, mix together the almond milk, maple syrup, ginger, cinnamon, nutmeg and salt. Pour in the cubed bread and coat it with the milk mixture. Set this aside as well.

3. Lightly grease the bottom of the slow cooker with butter. Slowly pour in a half of the milk and bread mixture into the pot then spoon one half of the banana mixture on top of it. Repeat the same order of layering.

4. Cover the pot and set the temperature to high. Cook the bread pudding for an hour and 45 minutes. Once the pudding is firm, turn off the slow cooker and serve it while it's hot.

Sliced Pears with Gooey Butterscotch Sauce

Preparation time: 10 minutes

Cooking time: 1 hour 10 minutes

Number of servings: 4

Ingredients:

- 2 apples, cored and sliced

- 2 ¾ cup butterscotch chips

- 1 tablespoon rum

- ½ cup evaporated milk

- ½ cup finely chopped almonds

Directions:

1. Place the milk and butterscotch chips in a slow cooker, cover it and cook on low heat for 1 hour. Stir the butterscotch sauce every 15 minutes.

2. After an hour, turn off the slow cooker. Add the rum and chopped almonds into the butterscotch and mix well. Pour the prepared butterscotch in a sauce bowl.

3. Arrange the apple slices on the sides of a serving dish. Place the butterscotch sauce at the middle or dunk a few pieces of fruit into the sauce. Serve immediately.

Homemade Chocolate Fudge

Preparation time: 5 minutes

Cooking time: 8 hours 10 minutes

Number of servings: 5

Ingredients:

- ¼ cup coconut milk
- 2 ½ cup dark chocolate chips
- ¼ cup raw honey
- 1 teaspoon vanilla extract
- Pinch of sea salt

Directions:

1. Place the milk, chocolate chips, honey, vanilla and salt in a slow cooker and mix well.

2. Cover the pot and set the temperature to low. Cook the fudge for 2 hours but do not stir it.

3. After 2 hours, turn off the slow cooker and uncover it. Lightly stir the fudge then leave it to cool for 3 hours.

4. Once the fudge has reached room temperature, use a wooden spoon to beat it for 10 minutes. Pour the fudge into a greased dish, cover it with plastic wrap then place it in a freezer for 3 hours.

5. Slice the chocolate fudge into squares before serving.

Slow Cooker Caramel Apples

Preparation time: 15 minutes

Cooking time: 1 hour

Number of servings: 6

Ingredients:

- 6 red apples, preferably Fuji or Gala variants

- 2 cups caramel candy cubes

- ¼ cup water

- Pinch of salt

- Popsicle sticks and wax paper

Directions:

1. Wash the apples and remove the stems. Pierce a popsicle stick halfway through each of the apples. Set this aside.

2. Place the caramel candies, salt and water inside a slow cooker. Cover it and cook the caramel on high for one hour.

3. Turn off the slow cooker and uncover it. Dip each apple into the caramel sauce, let the excess drip and place it on a sheet of wax paper to cool.

Chapter 16: Savory Dips, Sauces and Side Dishes Prepared With a Slow Cooker

Slow-cooked Caramelized Onions

Preparation time: 15 minutes

Cooking time: 5 hours

Number of servings: 4

Ingredients:

- 6 white onions, chopped into thin slices

- 1 teaspoon salt

- 2 tablespoons olive oil

- 1 teaspoon sugar

Directions:

1. Place the onions inside a slow cooker and add in the salt, sugar and olive oil.

2. Cover the pot and set the temperature to low. Leave the onions to cook for 5 hours.

3. Enjoy this sweet side dish with burgers, barbecued ribs or pulled pork sandwiches.

Gluten Free Marinara Sauce

Preparation time: 30 minutes

Cooking time: 10 hours

Number of servings: 15

Ingredients:

- 5 pounds chopped tomatoes

- 8 garlic cloves, chopped

- 3 onions, chopped

- ½ cup chopped fresh basil

- 1 cup chopped carrots

- ½ cup chopped fresh parsley

- ½ teaspoon cayenne pepper

- ½ cup olive oil

- 1 tablespoon sea salt

Directions:

1. Place the tomatoes, garlic, onion and carrots in a slow cooker.

2. Add in the basil, parsley, pepper, olive oil and sea salt and mix well.

3. Cover the pot and set the temperature to low. Cook the sauce for 10 hours and use a hand blender to mash up the tomatoes inside the pot.

4. Cool down the sauce and pour it into sterilized jars. Freeze the marinara sauce for a longer shelf life.

Spicy Tomato and Lentil Salsa

Preparation time: 10 minutes

Cooking time: 6 hours

Number of servings: 2

Ingredients:

- 1 ¾ cup chopped tomatoes
- ¼ cup green lentils
- ¼ cup gluten free salsa
- 3 garlic cloves, minced
- 1 red onion, chopped
- 2 teaspoons chili powder
- ¼ teaspoon ground cumin
- 1 teaspoon honey

Directions:

1. Place the tomatoes, lentils, salsa, garlic, onion, chili powder, cumin and honey in a slow cooker and cover it with a lid.

2. Set the temperature to low and cook the sauce for 6 hours.

3. Serve this dip with gluten free chips or crackers.

Cheesy Artichoke Dip

Preparation time: 15 minutes

Cooking time: 1 hour

Number of servings: 4

Ingredients:

- 2 cups chopped artichoke hearts, rinsed and drained
- 1 cup chopped spinach
- ½ cup sour cream
- ½ cup plain yoghurt
- 5 garlic cloves, minced
- 2 cups shredded Parmesan cheese

Directions:

1. Place the artichoke and spinach inside the slow cooker.
2. Pour in the sour cream, yoghurt, cheese and garlic. Mix the ingredients together.
3. Set the cooker's temperature to high and cook the dip for an hour.
4. Pour the dip in a bowl and serve with sliced carrots, cucumbers or gluten free crackers.

Slow Cooker Cranberry Sauce

Preparation time: 10 minutes

Cooking time: 4 hours

Number of servings: 8

Ingredients:

- 900 grams fresh cranberries

- 450 grams red apples, peeled, cored and sliced

- 1 cup honey

- 4 teaspoons cinnamon powder

- ½ cup fresh orange juice

Directions:

1. Place the apples, orange juice, cinnamon powder and cranberries in a slow cooker and cover it.

2. Set the crock pot's temperature to high and cook the fruits for 4 hours.

3. After 4 hours, allow the fruit mixture to cool then pour it into a blender. Puree the fruits completely then mix in the honey.

4. Pour the sauce in a serving bowl or store it in the freezer inside mason jars

Healthy Mock Mashed Potatoes

Preparation time: 10 minutes

Cooking time: 5 hours

Number of servings: 4

Ingredients:

- 1 cup almond milk

- 2 cups water

- 1 cauliflower cut into florets

- 5 garlic cloves

- 1 bay leaf

- 1 tablespoon gluten free butter

- 1 teaspoon salt

Directions:

1. Place the florets inside the slow cooker. Add in the salt, water, garlic cloves and bay leaf.

2. Cover the pot and cook for 5 hours on low temperature.

3. After 5 hours, remove the bay leaf and garlic cloves. Add in the butter and allow it to melt.

4. Mash the cauliflower mixture with a hand blender or a potato masher. While mashing, slowly pour the milk to make the

mixture creamier. The final product of this side dish should be similar to the texture of creamy mashed potatoes.

Slow Cooker Sausage Dip

Preparation time: 10 minutes

Cooking time: 25 minutes

Number of servings: 20

Ingredients:

- 600 grams spicy pork sausage, casing removed
- 1 ½ tablespoon olive oil
- 2 cups chopped tomatoes
- 1 tablespoon chopped green chilies
- 1 cup cream cheese

Directions:

1. Heat the olive oil in a large skillet over medium heat. Add the pork sausage stuffing and sauté until golden brown. Drain the excess oil from the meat and place it inside the slow cooker.

2. Add the cream cheese, tomatoes and green chilies into the sautéed sausage and cover the pot.

3. Set the temperature to medium heat and cook the dip for 25 minutes while stirring constantly. Serve immediately.

Sweetened Cream of Corn

Preparation time: 10 minutes

Cooking time: 3 hours

Number of servings: 12 servings

Ingredients:

- 1 ½ cup cream cheese, cut into cubes
- 1 cup cottage cheese
- 6 cups frozen corn kernels
- ½ cup butter, cut into cubes
- 2 tablespoons honey
- 4 tablespoons milk
- 2 tablespoons water

Directions:

1. Place the cream cheese, cottage cheese, corn, butter, honey, milk and water in a slow cooker and mix well.

2. Cover the pot and set the temperature to low. Cook the corn mixture for 3 hours.

3. Mix the creamed corn evenly before serving it as a side dish.

Conclusion

I'd like to thank you and congratulate you for transiting my lines from start to finish.

I hope this book was able to help you know more about the Wheat Belly program, including its food list, health benefits and guiding principles that are all geared towards helping you lose weight and achieve optimum wellness and also to cook gluten free dishes with confidence and ease with the use of a reliable and efficient slow cooker.

By trying the wheat-free recipes in this book, it is expected that you are now comfortable with using healthier alternatives such as almond flour, flaxseeds and liquid stevia to create healthy and flavorful dishes. These recipes will let you enjoy great-tasting meals everyday while you are in a personal journey towards achieving a lighter and disease-free body.

The next step is to try preparing healthier dishes on a daily basis that will not only satisfy the palate but also help you and the family become healthier and happier. Always remember that a gluten free lifestyle will help you achieve total wellness, and what better way to balance your body and energy than by enjoying a slow-cooked meal.

It's time for you to transcend the written word and keep on fighting for what you want in life. Go out there and fight for what is yours!

I wish you the best of luck!

To your success,

John Web

Made in the USA
Middletown, DE
27 November 2018